FOOD FOR THOUGHT

FIND OUT HOW TO NOURISH YOUR BODY AND SPIRIT THROUGH
HEALTHY EATING AND BIBLE STUDY

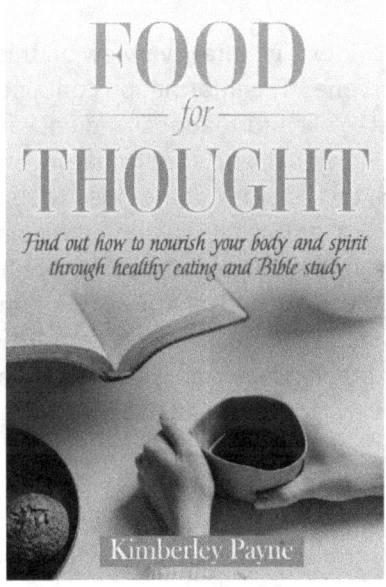

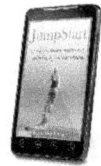 **Your Free Gift**

http://www.kimberleypayne.com/jumpstart/

JumpStart – Launch your journey to improve physical and spiritual fitness

JumpStart runs for 2 weeks, Monday to Friday, with the weekends off to catch up on any days missed, repeat challenges you like, or just take the time to rest and relax.

As prayer and Bible study are to the spirit what exercise and healthy eating are to the body Jump Start helps launch you into a healthy daily routine.

B – Bible Study
Each week, you're provided a new scripture to memorize. Each day, you're provided the same scripture verse but a different word is missing. This will help you to memorize one scripture by the end of the week.
E – Exercise
Each day, you're provided a short cardiovascular challenge and every Monday, Wednesday, Friday it'll be coupled with a simple strength training move to try.
E – Eating Healthy
Each day, you're provided a simple healthy eating challenge to encourage you to start thinking about what you're putting in your mouth.
P – Prayer
Each day, you're provided with a prayer that's based on the P.A.T.H. to prayer model where P stands for praise, A stands for admit, T stands for thank, and H stands for help.

Table of Contents

Introduction

Congratulations! You have made an important step towards a healthier you.

Food for Thought unites physical health and spiritual health to help you lose weight and develop a deeper relationship with God. You will gain insight into how to incorporate healthy eating and Bible reading into your daily routine.

God created you as a whole person, therefore, take care of your whole self, not just the individual parts. A healthy body gives you the energy and enthusiasm to carry out the purposes that God has for your life. Practicing healthy living glorifies God.

Feed your body + Feed your spirit

Healthy eating + Bible study

Just as eating healthy food nourishes your body, Bible study nourishes your spirit. Similarities between healthy eating and Bible study include:

- Healthy eating and Bible study are both activities that you need to do every day. They give strength and increase energy.

- There are different ways to perform each. You may eat healthy foods at home or at a restaurant. You may enjoy different food groups. Similarly, you may read your Bible at home or in a group. Also, many Bible versions are available to choose from.

- Both healthy eating and Bible study build healthy relationships. When eating, you can enjoy the company of your family and friends. When reading your Bible, you can build a healthier relationship with God.

- With a pure motive, both delight God.

Chapter 1: Feed your body

What it is

Then God said, "I give you every seed-bearing plant on the face of the whole earth and every tree that has fruit with seed in it. They will be yours for food."(Genesis 1:29)

Healthy eating nourishes your body. Eating well means eating a selection of foods that supply essential nutrients and energy.

Food touches every aspect of your life and affects how you feel. Healthy eating helps you to take care of yourself on the most basic level. God created a variety of foods that you can enjoy to meet the needs of your body. Food is a great source of energy and pleasure.

What it's not

Healthy eating does not need to be complicated. You do not need to cook extravagant meals or shop at specialty stores.

Eating well does not mean you have to give up any foods that you love. And it does not mean you have to start eating foods that you do not like. Everything you eat plays a part in keeping you healthy. Healthy eating means changing how much and how often you eat, not only what you eat.

Benefits of Healthy Eating

- Boosts energy level
- Improves concentration
- Reduces risk of cancer
- Reduces risk of obesity and diabetes
- Decreases risk of heart disease
- A pure motive delights God

Healthy eating gives you more energy for optimal physical and mental performance. You can reach a healthy weight and stay there without dieting.

Chapter 2: Healthy Eating Strategies that Work

Drink more water
Keep a water bottle on your desk, in your vehicle, and in the fridge. Use a larger glass than you typically use.

Eat breakfast
A wholesome breakfast not only fuels your muscles, but also prevents you from getting too hungry as the day progresses, at which point you simply do not care about what you eat and are likely to overeat. A good breakfast should include both carbohydrates and protein.

Try mini-meals
Switch from two to three large meals, to five or six smaller ones. More often, when you eat five or six times a day, you actually eat fewer calories than if you ate one or two huge meals.

Follow the 4-day rule
Try not to eat the same food within a four-day period. Enjoy many different kinds of foods to get all the energy and nutrients you need. You may even try a new drink or a new snack.

Spice it up
Focus on flavor. Add chilies, hot mustard and salsa to your meals or try flavorings such as lemon juice, herbs, and curry powders.

Make it easy

Buy vegetables and cut them for storage in the refrigerator, so the next time you want to grab something quick, it is already prepared.

Return to basics

Reduce the amount of processed foods you buy. If you really want to be healthy, get back to the basics with whole foods. Try to eat food the way God made it or as close to it as possible.

Pack a lunch

Bring your own foods as often as possible. A combination of carbohydrates and protein makes a great lunch.

Follow the 20-minute rule

Eat slowly. At meals, put down your fork. Give your brain the necessary 20 minutes to receive the signal that you have eaten your fill, so try to slow down the pace of eating.

Keep a food diary

A food diary helps to get a general idea of your daily calorie and food intake. It makes you accountable to yourself and more attentive to what you put in your mouth, when, and in what amounts. Keep a detailed food diary for seven to ten days.

Cut Back
Choose smaller portion sizes by cutting back a little at a time. Do not put more on the table than you want to eat at that meal and take away leftovers and unfinished dinners.

Eat mindfully
Eat sitting down and only in the kitchen or dining room. Focus on your food, not reading the newspaper or watching television.

Let go of extremes
Healthy eating should not be considered "on a diet" or "off a diet". Do not define yourself as a "success" or "failure" based on weight.

Use peace as your yardstick
Stop eating the food that you do not have peace about eating, "I know I shouldn't do this but…." When tempted, consider what is going on with you that is difficult to tolerate, or that you are trying to avoid. You need to be led by peace. If you do not have peace about it, do not do it.

Chapter 3: Healthy Eating Goal Planning

How do you get started?

Talk with your doctor
You should get medical clearance from your physician before making any significant changes in your diet.

An optimum diet takes into consideration many variables: calories, carbohydrates, protein, fats, food groups, and water.

Calories

Think of calories as a measure of heat that provides information about how much energy is contained in foods and how much energy the body expends.

Your optimal calorie intake needs depend on how much you weigh, how much muscle you have, and how much you exercise. For a woman who exercises moderately, 1800 to 2000 calories is a safe estimate. If you go below this amount, your metabolism (the rate at which you burn calories) may slow down.

Every 3500 calories consumed beyond your energy needs equals a gain of one pound of body fat. Therefore, a loss of 3500 calories is necessary to lose one pound of fat. However, short-term dieting does not work–it is not only about eating less but eating differently.

Every calorie you eat falls into one of three categories: carbohydrate, protein or fat.

Carbohydrate, protein, fat

A healthy weight is important, but the nutrients in the foods you eat really matter. Carbohydrate provides energy for the body. Protein builds and repairs body tissue. Fat protects internal organs and carries fat-soluble vitamins.

Fat contains twice the calories of protein and carbohydrates, so if you replace the fat with equal amounts of protein or carbohydrate you will save calories.

Generally speaking, the less processed or prepared your food, the lower the fat content.

Water

When thinking about your health, do not forget water. You may mistake thirst for hunger. If you drink first, you might not feel the need to eat. Lack of water can lead to dehydration and is a major trigger for daytime fatigue, headaches and irritability.

When the body gets the water it needs, it will function optimally. Water boosts your energy, suppresses appetite, increases short-term memory, prevents fluid retention,

improves concentration, maintains skin, relieves constipation and rids the body of waste.
You need to drink enough to keep your urine clear, light-colored and plentiful A dark, gold colour urine may mean you are dehydrated.

Remember to introduce changes slowly. Instead of trying to overhaul your lifestyle, take small steps. You have learned your eating habits over many years so take your time in changing them. Experiment with one thing at a time, so you will not feel overwhelmed. Set one nutrition goal every week, for example adding one fruit or vegetable serving each day.

Now it's your turn to make a list of goals that will help you improve your eating habits:

1.

2.

3.

Think about...

1. How many times a day do you usually eat, and at what times?

2. In the last year have you been eating the same amount of food/calories?

3. Are there small changes that you can incorporate into your grocery shopping?

4. How much time are you willing to commit to a healthy eating plan?

5. Write down your reasons for wanting to eat healthier.

Chapter 4: Feed your Spirit

What it is

Jesus answered, "It is written: Man does not live on bread alone, but on every word that comes from the mouth of God." (Matthew 4:4)

Bible study cleanses your spirit. The word Bible means "the books". It is the product of one Master Mind. The Bible itself internally claims to be God inspired and is something more than literature or history, it is God's Word. It is the best-selling book of all time.

You know that good nutrition is important to maintain healthy bodies. One of your best sources of spiritual nutrition is the Bible. Reading the Bible provides you with wisdom, instructions, and comfort – "nutrition" which helps you stay spiritually healthy. The Bible is food-for-thought and as with eating food, it is also important to "digest" God's Word.

What it's not

Bible study is not boring or irrelevant with over 40 different authors from all walks of life including priests, fishermen, prisoners and doctors. The writers came from a variety of locations and different eras. They used different writing styles including psalms, love songs, history, biography and letters.

Not just one big book, the Bible consists of 39 books in the Old Testament and 27 books in the New Testament for a total collection of 66 books. 400 years lapsed between the writing of the Old Testament and the New Testament. The writing of the Bible spanned over 1500 years, surviving cultural, geographic and political changes.

The Bible is not fable. The Bible is spiritually accurate with biblical prophecies fulfilled. Historical events and archaeology proved Bible truths.

Benefits of Bible study

- Provides insight and wisdom
- Details God's interaction with people
- Instills peace
- Promises hope for the future
- Builds a relationship with God
- A pure motive delights God

In the Bible, you will find guidance, promises and hope. All Scripture is useful for teaching, rebuking, correcting and training in righteousness. (2 Timothy 3:16)

Chapter 5: Bible Study Strategies That Work

Choose a Bible
There are many different versions of Bibles available.
Source one that you find comfortable reading. This book
quotes Scripture from the New International Version (NIV).
Some Bibles have added features such as introductions to
each book, character sketches, study notes and/or study
helps.

Read something each day
A little each day is better than a lot at once. In order to
devote time to reading this fascinating Book, it is helpful to
set aside the same time every day.

Expect God to reveal Himself
Pray a simple prayer and ask the Lord to change you and
reveal Himself to you through His Word. Begin by believing
that what you are reading is true. Read the Bible as if you
were reading a letter from someone who loves you.

Pick a study
There are many ways to study the Bible. You can visit a
library or Christian bookstore to choose from a variety of
helpful study guides. Many churches offer Bible studies for
small groups. Also, some Bibles even provide studies
within the text.

If you want a healthy spiritual life, you need to invest in it.
The Bible is food that helps you to grow strong and healthy
in your spirit.

Chapter 6: Bible Study Goal Planning

Can you remember a time when you may have had an intense yearning for something meaningful? A time when there was a constant nagging thought, "Is this as good as it gets?" A time when you sought not only a fleeting, happy moment but a true, pure and lasting joy?

Did the void feel insatiable? Did you turn to food to fill this void? If you feel like you still have this feeling than your relationship with food has to change. Instead of looking to food as your comforter look to the true Comforter. When you are feeling that emptiness turn to your Bible and read the Word. Only God can fill that empty space.

Instead of giving into the craving, realize what it is: a deep call to spend time with God, to learn about Him, and be with Him.

Reading the Bible is one way for you to do this. From the Bible you learn about God and can grow healthier each day.

Now it's your turn to make a list of goals that will help you improve your Bible study time:

1.

2.

3.

Think about...

1. How many days per week are you currently reading the Bible?

2. Have you ever participated in any type of Bible study?

3. At what time do you/would you usually read your Bible?

4. How much time are you able to commit to Bible study?

5. What will you have to give up to commit to reading the Bible?

Chapter 7: Test your Knowledge

Test your knowledge with these fill-in-the-blank questions.

Recipe for Success

1 Book

Reading the _____ provides you with wisdom, instructions, and comfort – "nutrition" which helps you stay spiritually healthy. The Bible is food-for-thought.

8 cups of water

When the body gets the water it needs, it will function optimally. Water boosts your _____, suppresses appetite, increases short-term memory, prevents fluid retention, improves concentration, maintains skin, relieves constipation and rids the body of waste.

4 tbsp of garlic, 4 pounds of chicken, 4 tsp of sesame seeds and 4 cups of apples

Try not to eat the same food within a _____-day period. Enjoy many different kinds of foods to get all the energy and nutrients you need. God created a variety of foods that you can enjoy to meet the needs of your body.

½ tsp each ground cumin and paprika

Focus on _____. Add chilies, hot mustard and salsa to your meals and try non-fattening flavorings such as lemon juice, herbs and curry powders.

1 cup each chopped onions and red bell pepper

Reduce the amount of processed foods you buy. If you really want to be healthy, get back to the basics with _____ foods. Try to eat food the way God made it or as close to it as possible.

Answers to fill-in-the-blanks:

Bible
Energy
Four
Flavor
Whole

Chapter 8: Action Plan

Recipe for Success

-Eat breakfast, lunch and dinner. A wholesome breakfast not only fuels your muscles, but also prevents you from getting too hungry.
-Read the Bible at breakfast, lunch and dinner. It will be easier to understand when you read smaller sections more often.

-Eat slowly. At meals, put down your fork. Give your brain the necessary 20 minutes to receive the signal that you have eaten your fill.
-Read the Bible slowly. Meditate and try to understand what it is you are reading.

-Choose smaller portion sizes by cutting back a little at a time.
-There are many Bible versions to choose from. Some Bibles have added features such as introductions to each book, character sketches, study notes and/or study helps.

-Eat sitting down and only in the kitchen or dining room. Focus on your food, not reading the newspaper or watching television.
-Read the Bible in a quiet room with no distractions.

-Stop eating the food that you do not have peace about eating. When tempted, consider what is going on with you that is difficult to tolerate, or that you are trying to avoid.
-Read the Bible to find peace.

Examples:

- I plan to cut fresh vegetables and keep in a container in the refrigerator
- I plan to participate in at least one Bible study each year
- I plan to keep a water bottle with me at all times
- I plan to read my Bible for fifteen minutes before the kids return from school

Your turn:

• I plan to

• I plan to

• I plan to

If you want a healthy spiritual life, you need to invest in it. The Bible is food that will help you to grow strong and healthy in your spirit. Use Jesus as your role model and the Bible as your guide.

In Closing

God's Word, the Bible, tells you that He created you. He loves you and He wants you to love yourself. You are beautiful. He has made everything beautiful (Ecclesiastes 3:11). I developed this program to help you feel good about yourself, no matter what your size. God wants you to be the most beautiful and useful person you can be. Your value is not found in physical appearance but in being a child of God.

Don't just endure life, enjoy it! You can enjoy healthy living – physically and spiritually. Taking care of your body and tending to your spirit adds joy to your life. One cannot be separated from the other. The body, mind and spirit are connected and reflected in your overall health.

There is much that demands your time. Time is a great sacrifice. Where do you want to spend your time? Whichever healthy activities you choose to continue with, make it a daily commitment. May God bless your journey towards improved spiritual and physical health.

For everything God created is good. (1Timothy 4:4a)

About the author

Kimberley Payne is a motivational speaker and writer. Her writing relates raising a family, pursuing a healthy lifestyle, and everyday experiences to building a relationship with God. Kimberley offers practical, guilt-free tips on improving spiritual and physical health. Visit her website www.kimberleypayne.com

Did you enjoy this book? Please take a moment to write a review. Share the blessings.

Books in the Fit for Faith Series

Fit for Prayer
Learn how to fit prayer and physical activity into your daily routine. The book unites physical health and spiritual health to help you lose weight and develop a deeper relationship with God.
Buy your copy! http://bit.ly/FitForPrayer

Food for Thought
Find out how to nourish your body and spirit through healthy eating and Bible study. Just as eating healthy foods nourishes your body, Bible study nourishes your spirit. You will learn practical suggestions and scriptural guidance to achieve your goals.
Buy your copy! http://bit.ly/Food-For-Thought

Flex your Spirit
Discover a new way to express yourself with God through journal writing and stretching. Learn how to recharge your physical and emotional health through stretching activities for your body and spirit.
Buy your copy! http://bit.ly/FlexYourSpirit

Fit for Faith – 7 weeks to improved spiritual and physical health combines all three books into **one workbook** plus adds health & fitness myths, a home fitness test, strength training and stretching exercises, and a food diary. The workbook also includes a 49-day plan to empower you to improve your spiritual and physical health!

Buy your copy today! http://bit.ly/FitForFaith7Weeks

Women of Strength – a devotional to improve spiritual and physical health includes a devotional article, question & answer, reflection, prayer, Bible truth, top tips, praise moves and a challenge to apply active living.

Buy your copy today!
http://bit.ly/WomenOfStrengthDevotional

Online Courses

www.kimberleypayne.com/e-courses/

Do you want to make the disciplines of exercise, prayer, healthy eating, Bible study, stretching and journal writing a part of your daily routine? All three books are also available as **virtual home-study courses.**

Home study
Watch the 7 video tutorials on your own time. Watch them all in a row, one a day or one a week. It's entirely up to you!

Spiritual component
Learn about prayer, Bible study, and journal writing to connect on a deeper level with God.

Physical component
Learn about healthy eating, cardio and strength training, and stretching exercises to incorporate into your day.

Support group
Ask questions, express concerns, and receive encouragement from other women.

Not sure if you want to commit to a full 7-module course? Visit www.kimberleypayne.com/free-programs to register!